Hope Stays Late

Hope Stays Late

Ned Haggard

April 8, 2020 —

For Karen Cox-Pedigo —

Class, character,
compassion, brilliance;
a special person

I am proud
and priviledged
to know —

Ned

Inland Lighthouse Publishing
Chicago, Illinois 60657

Inquiries may be addressed to the following:

Inland Lighthouse Publishing
Permissions Department
3023 N. Clark St.
#290
Chicago, Illinois 60657
Office: 708-595-3961
inlandlighthousepublishing@gmail.com

Any resemblance to any person, living or dead unless otherwise noted is purely coincidental. Any errors or omissions in the text or accuracy of the text are accidental. Considerable effort has been made by both the author and the publisher to ascertain accuracy and precision in any objective detail presented.

Library of Congress Cataloguing-in-Publication Data
Haggard, Ned
Hope Stays Late / By Ned Haggard
p. cm.
ISBN13: 978-0-9607780-1-0
1.   Title
LCCN: 2019900441

Cover Design:
Pamela Berns
Cover Layout Assistance:
Laura Coyle

Printed in the United States of America

First Edition, First Printing

Set in Garamond font typeface

Dedicated to Pamela K. Berns
Courage and Grace,
Determination and Faith
Incarnate...
"Pumpkin"

And to the memory of the late
Martin J. Rosenblum, Ph.D.

Do unto others as you would have them do unto you.

The Golden Rule

TABLE OF CONTENTS

ACKNOWLEDGMENTS

I wish to share my appreciation for the Introduction by Cressa Perish, M.D. and the back cover copy by Judith Paice, R.N., Ph.D.

INTRODUCTION

The words, "You have cancer," when uttered by one's physician, elicits an immediate response of fear for one's life, followed quickly by a chain of reactions including wondering how the dread disease chose them, how much longer their life will continue in the same or similar state, what has been accomplished in this life and what remains to be included in the future and even how it will end. All of these thoughts likely flash within a period of several minutes at most. Next comes sadness and often anger at the impact this unwelcome news will have on the plans in place for their lives and those close to them. Many times, what remains to be done is to take a deep breath, rally one's family and friends' support, choose a medical team and dive into the pool of Cancer treatment.

As a Family Practice physician for over 30 years, I have had the privilege of participating in the war on numerous and diverse diseases visiting many of my patients. I recall the day as an undergraduate when, in an epiphany, I first realized that we all, as members of the Human Race, share the same basic emotions and needs, regardless of our socio-economic, educational, geographic or philosophical backgrounds and that the same diseases can descend upon us, blind to our persons and our differences. Once the realization of our core common lot dawned on me, I was excited to join people as a physician assisting in their journeys toward health. Along the way, an invitation inside the deepest and most dear aspirations and, at times, the darkest fears of patients are a part of the journey shared by patient and chosen physician. It became clear early in my medical training that this sense of trust is built on those common experiences and must be treated as a rare and precious privilege. It gains great intensity shared with all those who offer support in the fight against Cancer.

The owners of the diagnosis of Cancer often find encouragement from their personal network and also from the full spectrum of the medical team, including smiles and thumbs up from the custodial staff, words of encouragement or a place to vent frustration. They find insight into the best way to manage their next round of chemo administered by an experienced nurse while securing the resources for ongoing financial support. Professionals ranging from a Social Worker to Treatment Team members and attendant physicians broaden each patient's understanding of the upcoming treatment protocol while encouraging each patient to ask all the questions stored up in anticipation of initial treatment or subsequent ones. As typical of Nature's synergism, family, friends and medical team members absorb energy in service of the renewal of effort while shooting the sometimes fierce rapids of treatment while keeping purpose with treatment. Determination is an accompanying aspect of continued experience along with the energizing experience of gratitude progressively and mutually generated and received among practitioners, patients, and support persons.

The miracle of Life, which is given to each of us is often taken for granted, as likely to be there tomorrow as is the bedside table when we awaken. We tend to plan our lives in chunks of time marked in minutes until the baby's nap is over and months until the next vacation and years until retirement brings the long-awaited time to kick up our feet and watch the birds in the backyard shake the seeds from the feeder to their companions on the ground. The precious seconds which comprise each of these chunks blur together and their significance is likewise unclear. The end of this gift of Life is usually not contemplated in all of this frenzied planning. Sometimes the gift is taken back abruptly with a fatal accident such as occurs on the highway when two vehicles collide or such as accidents within, as with a massive stroke or heart attack. These kind of final moments afford no opportunity to dispute the force which reclaims the gift. Occasionally, as is the case with Cancer, we are given a chance to rally all of our resources, either to mount the supreme fight to conquer the threatening robber of the gift of Life or to hold that gift before us and our loved ones to treasure and honor and to note the highlights before the light grows too dim.

In this thoughtful and sensitive collection of poems, *Hope Stays Late,* the accomplished poet, Ned Haggard appears to gather his vast talent and poetic tools to vividly capture the infinite range of emotions experienced by the people to whom the difficult news of Cancer is delivered. As well as the people who join that person along the remaining Life journey, whether to a field of Victory with a triumphant celebration and tenuous hope for the future or along a different path of honorable reflection regarding a Life whose future is to be taken away by the enemy known as Cancer and the recognition that the shortening of that Life, unfair and maddening as it is, does not subvert the value of that Life, however many days that Life has to tread on Earth.

Hope Stays Late is a delicate arrangement of glimpses into the true Miracle of Life in one of its greatest struggles, fighting serious disease, as exemplified in this case, Cancer.

Cressa Perish, MD
Family Practice Physician

Hope Stays Late

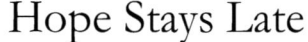

WARRIOR PHYSICIAN
(ONCOLOGY/HEMATOLOGY)

She has charm, buoyancy, energy; eyes (!)
that grasp, observe, eyes
that penetrate warmly, weighted, rarely
but sometimes piercing, even disdainful;
her air, assured; her mind,
incisive but too wise for easy
assumptions (a scientist-physician,
after all).
Underlying, an occasional
hint of superiority etched
of occupational default; but never
the empty vanity of
the shadow
narcissist....
Researcher and Practitioner,
Teaching Oncologist, she
has saved lives,
she
has scolded death,
brought it to its
knees, she
has delivered health or its best
approximation at mortality's
uncertain table;
a warrior physician
in the gnarly, mist veiled moor of
dread disease....

PATIENT

There is a presence to him, to
Many, perhaps nondescript,
but he is wiry, short, intelligently
focused. He chats with a nurse
In the waiting room, the air
of someone seeking
directions or explanation. On
his head he wears a skull
cap, religious or medical
I am not certain. It is a
loose mesh, white fabric
material. I have never before seen
any like it. He glances around
quickly, not wanting to be
distracted from
the exchange of words,
information, value. He reminds
me of Woody Allen in early
films in manner and
animation.

They part and walking, he
leaves mystery and
interest, an ethereal
imprint
lingering in the vacancy
he briefly occupied....

THE WAIT

Attractive, nearing early middle
age, she saw my noticing
her, seemed puzzled, her old
options evaded her. She looked away
uncertainly, sat down, straightened
her skirt, looked at the notification
vibrator in her hand, set it on the side
table. She looked sad, glanced
around at the old world as unfamiliar,
something freshly seen but opaque.
I wanted to comfort her, tell her I
liked her. She noticed me again,
glanced away reluctantly, unable
to judge. Her old responses no
longer dependably applied. Her
life now was a thin veil, no longer
something to cling to, no longer
something to depend upon, she
looked around anew trying to find
answers, reassurance, she glanced
at the wall behind the sitting people
facing her, awaiting their number
called, like her. She found nothing
in them but
a mirror. The wall provided no road
map, assurance escaped her, felt less
than
undependable. She was new to her
cancer, new to the reality of treatment,

Hope Stays Late

the equation: Successful or
failed, her life a thin veil, death
more real than her previous life had
informed her.

CIRCLING HOPE

The chemo bag hangs
from the medicine pole
feeding the arm of
the bright-eyed teenager who
chats sporadically with the
attendant nurse; she checks,
adjusts
the flow, moves the pole
slightly
closer. The teenager's
mother sits
quietly, reading the magazine
brought from the
lobby, glances up, observing
the nurse,
smiles briefly,
warmly at her
son, returns to her
reading. His girlfriend leans
forward in her seat,
gently pats his knee, smiling,
she takes his free hand, shares
a squeeze. His mother nods her
appreciation,
her approval; his father
calls from Scottsdale, away on
business.

Hope Stays Late

HOPE...

Differing ways of processing
their presence,
their emotions;
manifesting
styles
to ward off; perhaps as
talismans
of hope
concealing
fear,
concealing
despair,
prayer in
symbolizations and
gestures
wearing Hope!

SLOUCHING ONWARD

She lies half at
rest; half,
fringing sleep,
the light weave,
white blanket
over her, drawn
to her chin. Her
relative youth
(Late 30's, perhaps;
give, not take)
showing somewhat
bony faced,
somewhat gaunt;
her complexion
sallow, nearing
gray, nearing…

The attendant
blue frocked nurse,
young, focused,
dedicated in her
care adjusts
the IV
pole, attends
to her patient's
needs, efficiently,
quietly;
her deference to
her patient's lull
toward

7

Hope Stays Late

sleep apparent in her
studied
quiet; her patient's
demeanor
in rest,
peaceful; her patient's
knowing gently etched
in her
slight, journey-wise
smile. She rests, care
swaddling her....

CUSTODIAN

Cordial, knowing
The aging custodian
serves,
attentive to
whatever housekeeping
necessity at hand (empty
styrofoam cups left
on waiting room tables,
garbage to collect for
incinerator fates,
coffee to make,
water bottles to
replace, anon),
attentive to
those waiting for their names and
paging vibrators to be called
or sound; he greets the older
patients and companion visitors,
"Hello young man; good day, ma'am,"
continues on;
some smile
greeting in
return, some remain
focused within
waiting on destiny, unknown
fate....

MAKING PLANS

Chatting, the two patients
share experience,
share plans, while
their chemo drips across
distracted minutes,
unnoticed;
he intends to take
his granddaughter
to Hawaii; the
other intends to
write a book.... Their
progressively
drawn faces
keep their plans
as the hopefulness
of the living.

RESIDENT PSYCHIATRIST, MD, PhD

Gracious, accomplished, often
distracted between
patients
he assesses emotional
characteristics,
prescribes medication in service of
comfort with cancer,
in service of patient
ease, in service of
health, brings graciousness
to treatment and
for some,
eases mortality's
end.

YOUNG

Enthusiastically waiting,
legs crossed, slouched back
in the armchair
chatting
on her cell
like she's at
a coffeehouse
taking a call
or making one
from/to old
friends...

She is a patient;
Cancer.
She's young,
likely
early 20's...

Her number and first name
is called
by the Medical Aid
from the Treatment
Area
doorway...

"I have to go,"
she says,
hurries
toward the Aid who

holds her med order...

At night, alone,
she stares up at the ceiling
trembling....

SPIRALING YEARS & SWEET REMEMBRANCES

Chemo bag hanging, the
infusion pump
mid-medication IV pole
near armrest hand,
the man snores
somewhat softy; his
wife nearby, sitting leans
forward, smiles warmly a
hint of amusement in
her kindly focused, seeing
eyes, peering through years
of their lives shared
of their lives in common
of their lives: first kisses,
early dates, their marriage,
their children, one then
two, maybe more...
trials and successes;
her smiling sight betraying
vision; her eyes set
upon her husband,
seeing memories, fully alive as he
snores while his treatment
progresses....

DIGNITY

The tall, blue-black ink skinned, chemo
bald woman
apologizes for having
turned my seat-keeping
cap into a registration
clerk. "No problem,
ma'am, thank you
for turning it
in," I reply, awed,
startled, amazed. Within
the larger city
a stepped-on youth
seeking himself,
a Man!
serves up death
from the end of a trigger
pull gun,
not so sure from
the river red flow of blood;
a child dead in her
mother's crying aloud arms.
Adrenalin pumps.
He flees with his gang,
boasts new colors amid high fives,
those bullets do whiz,
I's a Man! The woman
rises awkwardly from her waiting room
armchair, her pager number
called out by the nurse's aide
smiling greeting at the treatment area

Hope Stays Late

doorway. The woman makes her
unsteady way toward her, her cane her
only support, smiles weakly,
greeting the nurse, keeps faith
while her disease relentlessly
tightens
her skin on her frail, failing
frame,
day-by-day,
knowing fully
her evermore visible
end, exuding an air of wry
irony, wearing
dignity's victory
before the face
of fate

RN, PhD (Hematology/Oncology)

Attentively searching she
observes,
relieves pain (her
specialty)
shares helpfulness
knowledgeably. She
challenges the subversiveness
of cancer. Engages it
head on with medicinal
astuteness, suggestions
to ease and
reassure
with the reality
of lab measured
promise....

TRADITION SETS FAITH'S TABLE

They were within and without
A part and apart,
unfamiliar. The Rabbi
the most at ease, years of gracious
authority sanctioned of G-d and
Abrahamic Tradition. His wife,
chatty and wary, engrained
of millennia of quiet, astute
surveillance, rooted in Exodus,
rooted in the undependability
of Diaspora, rooted in pogroms,
rooted in round ups and
Holocaust persecution. Rooted
in tunnels burrowed under borders
of hostile lands neighboring Israel.
This time, it is the unseen, the
threat of disease that
puts all on edge,
puts all on weary
guard; the Patriarch,
the Husband,
a young son, two
elder daughters,
all face a different
threat, without prejudice, not
rooted in tribal hatreds,
not rooted in Anti-Semitic bias
but rooted in physical cells and
the mystery of cellular
change, hope anchored

in calm and faith,
anchored in prayer,
anchored in appeal,
anchored in the inherent dignity of
"Rabbi."

CUTE BUT NOT ONLY....

Almost doll like, she sits, sight
inwardly focused, sight
withdrawn to mortal
possibilities, composed
yet preoccupied, her
long fingered hand
reaches to forehead,
she turns her head
into its touch; I
wonder to her memories,
does she wonder to the
dreams of her childhood?
To dresses and mud pies,
to running with the wind
during recess, squealing
delight with girlfriends,
to apprehensive reaching
for control via ignoring an
admiring boy, secretly
delighted but uncertain,
vulnerable in the newness
of his awareness of
her? I wonder, as she soldiers on
bravely
facing her
cancer, her beauty now early
middle aged mature yet
fresh.... Does she wonder and
recall the early days as though
just around the corner she

turned entering
the waiting room and
treatment? Neither hopeful
nor despairing? Her head
in poised hand speaks proverbial
volumes, a posture of one living
with hope and as of yet
unanswerable questions....

CLINICAL PSYCHOLOGIST, PhD

She listens attentively to
patients,
hears, commiserates,
suggests,
as cancer raises its
skirt displaying
the person
within the
pain of uncertainty
and fear,
hope and
despair.

CONTENTION AND RESPECT

Cancer treatment, high stress,
focused work; medical hierarchy,
working teams
occasional tension,
ego stress, varied
opinions generally
evaluated for worth,
integrated
for value,
for healing;
a team
sharing
respect, embracing
camaraderie in
the campaign; a
fierce war countering
cancer, serving
Life!

BITTER STREET

The curtain drawn separating patient
spaces, the IV pole
next
to the armchair
supports the chemo bag; medicinal drip
tubing runs to the young man's
arm, belies his silence. Days past
memories carry carefree
images of running with chums,
rollicking, yelling their nascent
ages. Leaving school for home, the
baseball practice over, spring
in the air, in their
steps, their near leaps of joy; his
girlfriend's touchdown proud,
twinkle star
eyes. He
does not return their
phone calls, does not answer
their text messages, emails, does not
open the door, erases
his sorrow with their messages, their
memories. Early 20's and wondering,
will he survive?
Will he die? If so, when? Too few moments
serve forgetfulness, too many
memories serve the
bitter swindle, the bitter street
betrayal; life, no longer
certain.

ADVANCED PRACTICE NURSE, PhD, MSN

Attractive with warm eyes
betraying sensitivity,
betraying recognition, awareness,
betraying attentiveness to patients and
others: spouses, friends,
relatives, significant
persons; she listens,
discerns, sometimes
kindly bemused (never
disregarding), supportive,
offering knowledge subverting
doubts, easing uncertainties,
relieving the pain and
fear of the worried,
relieving the pain of
caring companions; those
yearning for hope in the face of
the fickle potential of
cancer; not false,
nurturing, a soldier's firm
shoulder in the war on
malignancy's
savage randomness,
malignancy's dumb
indifference:
Nurse.

VOLUNTEER

Efficient, walking retired miles
serving
patients, the cancer center,
the doctors, the nurses,
assorted staff; congeniality
wrapped in
warmth greets,
chats
in passing
recognizing, those not
dead
are living,
recognizing fate
is always opaque
until revealed,
recognizing caring
matters, recognizing
busy practice
is sometimes curt,
directive, seemingly impersonal;
volunteers bring
devotion alive
with the value
of touch, the
value of a recognition nod,
the value
of a smile.

EMBRACE

Young, spirited and in a tender exchange
of words, the couple looks on
one another with the casual ease of
confident age. The young woman,
stunning with alabastrine complexion,
a healthy blush of shapely, springtime
flesh, appreciatively shares her sight,
smiles a bright red lipstick smile;
her husband reflects her bright composure,
her hopeful winsomeness,
holds her coat; next, her chemo bald head
is covered beneath her crimson,
knit cap. They walk, chatting lightly,
holding hands, from the treatment
center toward the elevator bank,
toward another
promising day...

YEARS POOLED IN LOVING EYES

Years pooled in loving eyes,
loving sight, as her
husband sits,
snoring, neither loud
nor soft
sees children and
dreams lost and
found as he snores
as she sees
the years together
a good man, indeed
a good father, too;
the apartment,
later a house,
and then another,
larger as their family
grew
until they grew to move
into their own
and now a condo
just enough room,
she smiles the years
she sees: their private
memory film of
life as he snores
the chemo needle in
his arm (alive, invisibly
arm-in-arm) ....

CLOSING TIME

Tastefully, nondescript, institutional décor
cool, not quite cold
waiting area
busy an hour earlier with
patients holding
pagers, awaiting nurse assistants
stepping from set back
entry ways calling
their pager numbers, red lights
concurrently flashing the symbolic,
"Next." The vacuous waiting
area all but vacant now,
medical shifts over, patients
admitted, or returning home,
or having drawn their last
malignancy breath with
sheet drawn over
their reclined remains,
the Aredia treatment
bags still hanging from
the IV pole stand in reminder
of their last resilience
bygone, hope left behind before
eternity's mystery;
awaiting the quiet transport to
the hospital morgue and
the helpless sighs and tears
of those not yet
gone, not yet breath abandoned,
not yet beyond inevitably

Hope Stays Late

transient hope...

Closing time....

DREAMS COME TRUE
(More and more often, they do)

A long road, with anxiety,
fear, courage and worry:
Will I Live, or
Die? Will I know
pain I can
hardly bear?
Or will it be a
pillow down
dream drifting to
the arms of
malignancy's end,
eternity? Neither,
you say? Oh, Doctor,
Thank you, Thank you,
Thank you! Remission, you
say. Truly? Oh,
never a more beautiful
word, it rings like a church
Bell, it rings in
Christmas come, early, on
time
or late, it matters not (the
Greatest gift of
all); it rings the echo of
Miracle's chimes….
Remission has
Arrived!

WARRIOR PHYSICIAN #2

She speaks softly, her focus
fixed on the patient; a key
marker has risen.
She speaks reassurance,
lends conviction in
manner and comment;
"We are revising your
treatment, I am only being
cautious." Her patient
eases into a newly relaxed
posture, seated with
an IV secured in her elastic
bandage wrapped
arm. Her physician's parting words
keep
the patient
like an infant
cozied in a warming quilt;
departing, the physician's
steady steps
lend a calm, certain
focus as she walks
to the next patient in
her ongoing war
on cancer.

ABOUT THE AUTHOR

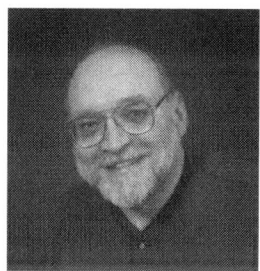

Ned Haggard has lived a far-ranging life with writing often at the core of his explorations of varied human experience here and abroad. He did a Cultural Exchange to Oxford University and studied Creative Writing - Poetry at Harvard University. Now retired, he held editorial and marketing positions in the bookselling/publishing industry. His writing, primarily neo-objectivist imagist poetry, but also short stories and an excerpt from a forthcoming mystery, has appeared in numerous literary journals and several anthologies. He is the author of The Weave of the Sea, a collection of poetry and was the founder and publisher of Lakes & Prairies: A Journal of Writing, a publication that gained the attention of Diane Wakoski, Denise Levertov, Allen Ginsberg and singer-songwriter-author, Leonard Cohen. He currently is the Review Editor for Chicago Life magazine. His poem "Mellow" was delivered, along with the work of other poets, to the Trump White House (The poem is included in the author's website: www.nedinwriting.com).

Made in the USA
Monee, IL
25 November 2019

17393198R00032